Weight loss and you: how to start losing weight

Lydia Miller

Table of Contents

Introduction

With handled food varieties that are high in fat promptly accessible now adays, it seems like many individuals have wound up expanding. Actually, the level of people suffering from corpulence has been on the ascent as of late. While a portion of these individuals are nonchalant about the need to shed pounds, others have ended up looking for items for weight misfortune. There are different justifications for why people want to get more fit, one of which would be because of worry for their wellbeing. Because of different wellbeing alarms and reports in newspapers,people are now more aware that being obese can actually be bad for their bodies.As such, they might need to shed over abundance pounds before they have experience wellbeing problems and it is too late.

The market for such items and administrations has developed, with weight reduction helps, for example, slimming programs, thinning enhancements, and pills that should confine your body's admission of carbohydrates professing to have the option to assist buyers with achieving their fantasy weight. There are also those who choose to take a more extreme measure by going under the knife to have the size of their tolerates precisely decreased. With the various choices we have today, certain individuals are now starting to believe that there are quick and speedy methods for shedding pounds. Nonetheless, this may not necessarily be great for your body.

There are numerous who have decided to adhere to the more customary techniques for getting thinner - to diet and to work out. Notwithstanding, with regards to consuming less calories, there are such countless decisions you can choose from that you might wind up confounded concerning which diet program will be best for you.You might try and contemplate whether diet programs are successful in assisting you with shedding pounds. If these are some of the inquiries that you as of now have at the forefront of your thoughts, then you can definitely relax!

How Can Weight Loss Benefit You

There are numerous ways of losing weight. A portion of the strategies that individuals use to lose weight include practicing and confining their eating regimens to accomplish the best weight reduction results. As such, individuals who might want to accomplish their fantasy weight celebrate with the different options available.

Be that as it may, even with these weight reduction choices accessible, certain individuals are as yet inadequate with regards to the will to work towards their fantasy weight. Rather than battling the fat, they just acknowledge their current weight and fail to address it. This might be on the grounds that they know nothing about how putting effort and being inspired to get thinner will help them to accomplish different advantages for their body.

Assuming you're among these individuals who have abandoned getting in shape, you ought to consider these benefits before halting your battle against excess weight and inches.

With regards to shedding pounds, medical advantages are on the first spot on the list of justifications for why you should buckle down. By shedding pounds and not being large, you will also have the option to decrease your risk of getting serious illnesses later on. For example, individuals who have abundance weight usually foster diabetes because of an expanded degree of glucose. The issue with this condition is it very well may be hard to treat and would require ordinary insulin infusions in order to control this medical condition.If the illness worsens, the patient may even need to undergo dialysis.This is on the grounds that diabetes can keep your kidneys from sifting the blood in your body, causing waste in your body to enter your circulatory system. As your kidneys can't work well,dialysis will turn into a basic piece of your life as it will finish the work that your kidneys can no longer perform.While you maybe prompted by your illness to keep a watchful eye on your diet

what's more, work out, it might simply be excessively late, as you might need to battle with your condition for your entire life.

Weight reduction additionally can help your body maintainits balance. Having a weighty body may make individuals move at a more slow speed and even lose their equilibrium from time to time.When you have an enormous weight, you will have more prominent latency. All things considered, your body will find it hard to move, particularly when it is sudden. Be that as it may, in the event that you can shed pounds, you will feel much lighter and more nimble. This will be useful for you, particularly in the event that you are consistently on the go.Balance will not be a problem anymore so you can move at a faster pace than before.

At last, individuals who get thinner will likewise end up setting aside cash simultaneously. This benefit might come in various ways. At the point when you get more fit, you are less inclined to develop diseases like diabetes or heart issues. In that capacity, you will actually want to save the money needed for hospitalization, medicine and different medicines, for example, treatment meetings and dialysis.

Aside from medical clinic charges, you may likewise observe that looking for garments is currently simpler and cheaper with your new estimations. This is on the grounds that when you get thinner, you won't need to shop at stores that work in hefty size garments. All things considered, you will actually want to just head on down tothe closest shopping center to select new garments for yourself. Shedding creeps from your body will help you find clothing that will fit you at affordable costs.

In that capacity, weight reduction is only useful for yourself and you can do it with the assistance of exertion and motivation.Start planning your weight loss program today to experience these benefits.

Things You Should Know Before Starting Any Weight Loss Program

Weight reduction has turned into a first concern for the overwhelming majority people nowadays. Certain individuals would like to accomplish this exclusively for stylish purposes, while others have been affected by medical statistics. For one's purposes, serious clinical issues like diabetes and heart issues are beginning to become progressively common among individuals who are late 20s up to mid 30s. In that capacity, many have started on weight misfortune programs to avoid having these health problems.

At the point when you are searching for the right get-healthy plan, it's imperative for you tobe arranged and have sensible assumptions for it. Coming up next are a portion of the things you should know before choosing and beginning your weight loss program.

Not all weight loss programs will work of everyone

Everybody is unique. Accordingly, get-healthy plans won't significantly affect everyone,especially since there will be contrasts in metabolic rates and the singular's responsibility tothe program. While you can think about how the program has helped other people,you ought to be ready for results that are unique. In the event that you are searching for a decent weight loss program for yourself, you won't just have to do explore, yet additionally utilize your feeling of judgment so as to keep away from frustrations.

Weight loss is achievable with diet and exercise

There are alot of diet programs that might be able to give you good results. Nonetheless, for effective weight reduction, counts calories are not sufficient.The truth is that eating regimen and exercise complement each other. Consequently, other than limiting what you eat, you ought to likewise invest energy doing exercises everyday for remarkable weight loss.

Motivation is key

Many individuals start and quit their health improvement plan when they have lost interest or reached a plateau. Actually the majority of these people simply come up short on inspiration to get in shape. They easily surrender following a few days of doing the program in light of eagerness. They may have found the best program for them yet all that will go to squander by surrendering in the program.Set your motivation and be patient instead of rushing to get results.

Consult your physician for advice.

Certain individuals might hurry into get-healthy plans without talking with their doctors. Accordingly, they end up not obtain the ideal outcomes and may try and acquire wounds or clinical issues. In the event that it ispossible, you ought to have your wellbeing assessed by your essential consideration supplier before taking part in any program. Doctors will suggest a health improvement plan, comprising of both diet and work out, which will be reasonable for your requirements and custom-made by your capacities. This will allow you to achieve the results you desire without putting a strain on your body.

With these snippets of data, you are currently prepared to leave on your weight reduction journey.When you have the perfect proportion of exertion and inspiration, you can achieve your desired weight loss.

Do Weight Loss Diet Programs Really Work?

The significance of weight reduction has been recognized by numerous people around the world.The fixation on getting thinner has made business people and organizations come up with different approaches that will help people to lose weight efficiently.

While every one of these eating routine projects guarantee to be successful, as a shopper, you ought to be meticulous with subtleties when you are thinking about such items. This is on the grounds that the web might be quite deceiving in some cases. Assuming you see positive tributes for their things on the item's website,you can not decide whether the tributes are genuine. Regardless of whether the weight reduction diet programs are powerful, the outcomes that you see might be not the same as what you anticipate. As such,here are somethings that will prepare you in terms of diet programs'effectiveness.

Results of diet programs may vary

Diet projects will be successful, yet results will be different for people. Some might lose anenormous measure of weight while others may essentially have humble results.A number of factors contribute to this situation, for example, metabolic rates and how committed are the people to the diet program. On the off chance that you have high metabolic rates, you will find it simpler to get in shape as compared to people with lower metabolic rates.Apart from the physical factors,varying levels of commitment to the program likewise lead to various outcomes. Some will zero in on the program by following it rigorously while others might wind up surrendering to the allurement of food varieties that are not diet-accommodating.

Work out

Individuals would believe that diet alone can assist them with getting the best results.The truth is you'll track down that even the developers of these programs will still recommend daily short exercise sessions.

In fact, you'll find that some of them would even indicate specific amount of time you should use working out and the types of exercise you should do. For example, they might recommend users to do 30 minutes of aerobic exercises every other day to achieve better results. As such,diet and exercise should go hand in hand.

Different states of health

Diet programs will usually require specific food types or products which are to be eaten as partof the weight loss program. However, there are some of the food requirements that may not be suitable for an individual. This is where consulting with a health expert will be helpful. If you would like take part in a diet program, you must first consult your primary care provider and tell them the foods that it may require. They'll check out your current health state through your regular checkups. Once they approved of the program, you can start on it. You may also ask for suggestions on which program you should participate in so that you will be able to go on a diet that suits you best.

Conclusion

All in all, diet projects can be powerful for weight reduction, however the progress of such programs will rely upon certain elements. It's energetically prescribed for you to have your well being assessed before trying out any program in the market so that you will be able to get the best results.

While you might be quick to shed off those over abundance pounds, you ought to just do so steadily. There are numerous who decide to adhere to count calories programs, whether it is about just eating chosen foods, keeping your calorie intake below a certain amount or eating less.However,there are also some who have made consumes less calories a stride excessively far by not eating enough or having adequate nutrients and nutrients.As such,not only will you be unable to enjoy the positive benefits of losing weight,you may even find your health breaking down!

For sound weight reduction, you ought to continuously get things done with some restraint, be it practicing or dieting.Of course, you can enroll the assistance of an expert specialist who will exhort you on what you should do. You should trust yourself and consistently accept that you will be capable to lose weight successfully.

With these tips in mind,you will definitely be ready to lose weight and enjoy a healthier life!

www.ingramcontent.com/pod-product-compliance
Lightning Source LLC
Chambersburg PA
CBHW081510250726
48662CB00021B/3195